OSTEOARTHRITIS

==========

Control It
or
It Will Control You

RON KNESS

Copyright © 2016 Ron Kness

All rights reserved.

ISBN-13: 978-1533521590

ISBN-10: 153352159X

Contents

Disclaimer 3

Introduction 4

Chapter 1 – Preventing and Managing Arthritis 7

    What Is Arthritis? 7

Chapter 2 – Getting Enough Exercise/Physical Activity 10

Chapter 3 – Using Common Sense In Relation to Working Out ... 13

Chapter 4 – The Best Workouts For Those With OA 16

Chapter 5 – Maintaining A Healthy Weight 19

Chapter 6 – Eating A Healthy, Balanced Diet 23

Chapter 7 – Trying An Anti-Inflammatory Diet 26

    Best Foods to Eat 28

    Foods To Avoid 32

Chapter 8 – Improving Joint Mobility And Stability 35

Chapter 9 – Using Assistive Devices 38

Chapter 10 – Using Complementary And Alternative Therapies ... 41

Chapter 11 - Herbs and Supplements 44

Chapter 12 – Managing Symptoms, Such As Pain, Stiffness and Swelling 46

Chapter 13 – Over The Counter Medications 49

Chapter 14 – Prescription Medications 51

Chapter 15 – Maintaining A Positive And Healthy Mindset............ 53

Chapter 16 – Considering Surgical Options..................................... 56

Conclusion 58

Resources 60

Other Senior Health and Fitness Books by This Author 61

About The Author.. 68

Disclaimer

Use caution when beginning a new health program.

Not all recommendations are suitable for everyone. This publication is for informational purposes only and is not intended as medical advice. Medical advice should always be obtained from a qualified medical professional for any health conditions or symptoms associated with them.

Every possible effort has been made in preparing and researching this material. We make no warranties with respect to the accuracy, applicability of its contents or any omissions.

Check with your doctor before you begin.

Introduction

There are literally dozens of diseases that have arthritis as one of the main symptoms of the disease. However in this book, we focus on one of the most common in aging adults – osteoarthritis.

It is also referred to as degenerative joint disease, wear and tear arthritis, or degenerative arthritis and affects about 27 million adults in the US. It can affect any joint of the body but is more prevalent in the hips, neck, knees, lower back, and the tiny bones of the hands and feet.

The occurrence of arthritis is caused by degeneration of the cartilage that normally covers the ends of the bone and allows for smooth motion of the joints. Common symptoms include joint pain, swelling, and stiffness of the joints.

My doctor classified it as a "wear and tear" condition. I guess he didn't want to use the word "degenerative". For me (as it does for most people having it) happens over time and there wasn't really anything I could have done to prevent it, except to maybe change to a different line of work – one less demanding on joints.

Early in my career, I was in auto and truck mechanics meaning I used my hands a lot, spent time bent over working on engines, etc., so my joints got a lot of use and probably abuse, but I didn't know that at the time.

Also because of the work I was in, I have had several small joint injuries along the way all adding to the issues I now have with osteoarthritis according to my doctor.

However, since being diagnosed and struggling to manage the symptoms – there isn't a cure short of joint replacement and I'm not there yet - I have been on a mission to learn how to control it and minimize its effects.

Osteoarthritis is a chronic, that is, long-term disease without any known cure at the present time. It affects more than 27 million in the US, and can occur at any age, from childhood through to one's senior years.

Most cases of OA occur after age 45, making it a disease commonly associated with growing older.

With Americans living longer than ever before, the number of cases of arthritis is bound to increase in the next couple of decades.

As something I have been diagnosed with and lived with for a number of years, osteoarthritis (OA) is a topic near and dear to me, but not by my choice. Out of necessity, over the years I have learned to live with it and will share some things that have worked for me in hopes they may help others afflicted with it too.

The main consideration is not just duration of life, but quality as well. The longer a person can stay mobile, the more independent they will be, and generally in better health, with less pain.

If you are ready to do more for the benefit of your bone and joint health, or have started to feel the pain and stiffness of OA, there are a number of strategies proven effective in preventing and managing OA. In this guide, we will explore a range of safe, natural options supporting healthy joints, many of them that have worked for me.

Chapter 1 – Preventing and Managing Arthritis

While arthritis in general can happen at any age, and can run in families, there are a number of ways to prevent arthritic symptoms and manage OA long-term without suffering from too much pain and disability. As with all chronic conditions, it is a case of being vigilant and assessing what works well, then doing more of it.

What Is Arthritis?

Arthritis is a condition in which the joints are inflamed. You can have just one joint involved in arthritis or many joints afflicted with the condition. Arthritis can be unilateral and affect just one side of the body or bilateral, affecting joints on both side of the body.

Arthritis has many causes. Some types of arthritis are secondary to eating foods that allow crystals to develop in the joints, resulting in joint pain, redness, and swelling of the joint. Gouty arthritis is an example of this.

Arthritis can also be caused by wear and tear on the joints or overuse of the joints. This is usually how people get osteoarthritis, which affects both large and small joints. Some people get arthritis from autoimmune diseases in which antibodies are made by the immune system that attack joint tissues, resulting in joint inflammation, swelling, and chronic joint pain.

Typical symptoms of arthritis include pain in the joints, redness, and swelling near the inflamed joint, joint stiffness, and an inability to move the joint without experiencing pain. As mentioned, medications can be given to control these symptoms; however, there are dietary changes you can make that can also reduce inflammation and can relieve joint pain without having to take medications to control the symptoms.

Prevention, and long-term management of OA can be pictured as a multi-pronged attack plan. Success strategies include:

- Getting enough exercise/physical activity
- Using common sense in relation to working out
- Maintaining a healthy weight
- Eating a healthy diet
- Trying an anti-inflammatory diet
- Improving joint mobility, flexibility and stability
- Using assistive devices

- Using complementary and alternative therapies, including herbs and supplements
- Managing symptoms, such as pain, stiffness and swelling, including the use of over the counter medications
- Prescription medications
- Maintaining a positive and healthy mindset
- Considering surgical options if you are not getting enough relief from the other methods or the damage is just too severe.

We will discuss each of these in turn on the pages below.

Chapter 2 – Getting Enough Exercise/Physical Activity

One of the most beneficial ways to manage OA is to keep moving in order to avoid the pain and stiffness associated with this type of arthritis. Regular physical activity promotes strong bones, muscles, joint and ligaments and increases flexibility. These in turn contribute to a healthy, stable joint that will be much less prone to injury.

Solid core muscles can also prevent back pain and back injury when performing routine tasks such as lifting moderately heavy weights like groceries or 40 lb. bags of salt for the water softener.

If you have OA already, the thought of exercise may make you cringe. Your joints already hurt enough. The truth is that one of the best ways to relieve the pain is to move around. Stiffness leads to pain, and pain can lead to inactivity. Inactivity leads to stiffness, and stiffness leads to pain. Soon you are caught in the vicious cycle of OA pain.

Yes, it may hurt to move around, but too much rest will only lead to more pain. Striking a balance is the best way to stay mobile well into your senior years. Studies show that simple activities like walking around the neighborhood or taking a fun, easy exercise class can reduce pain and help maintain or achieve a healthy weight. I have found that exercising in a pool helps reduce the pain because there is low to no impact on joints, especially the knees.

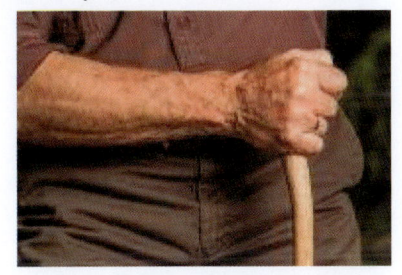

Strengthening exercises build muscles around OA-affected joints, easing the burden on those joints and reducing pain. Range-of-motion exercise helps maintain and improve joint flexibility and reduce stiffness. Aerobic exercise helps to improve stamina and energy levels and also help to reduce excess weight. Yoga is a great form of exercise that helps increase flexibility and is easy on the joints. Many yoga studios have classes just for those with arthritis.

If you have not be working out for a while, you should first speak with your doctor to determine whether or not you are well enough to work out, and if there are any limitations to your activities. They might provide guidelines, or refer you to a physical therapist or sports medicine therapist.

The next step is to start slowly, using common sense in relation to working out. Let's look at this topic in the next chapter.

Chapter 3 – Using Common Sense In Relation to Working Out

One of the main causes of OA is wear and tear on the joints. This may not seem like a big deal when you are younger, but repetitive workouts and injuries can have serious consequences over time. Working a couple of sessions with a personal trainer can teach you about proper form in the gym so you will not injure yourself using any of the equipment, and to gradually ease into any exercise program.

The most common area affected by OA is the knee. It is a complex joint that can easily be injured through contact sports such as soccer and American football, and through high-impact, high-risk sports such as skiing and snowboarding. Repetitive activities like jogging, cycling and spinning can all lead to wear and tear over time, especially if you are not observing the proper posture and form or overdoing things every day.

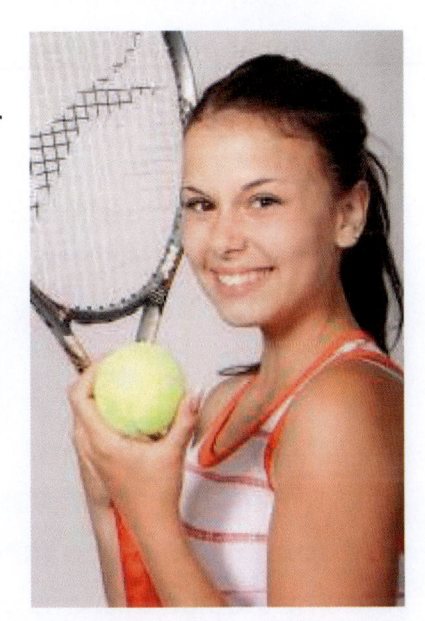

Men are most commonly affected by OA of the knee through sports injuries, or the results of vehicle-related accidents. These can happen at any age, but are more likely to happen as we get older and lose strength and muscle mass. We lose muscle mass at the rate of 1 pound per year once we hit 40. This may not sound like much, until you consider that by the time you reach 80, if you have not been paying attention to building muscle, you will be only half as strong as you were.

Note that losing a pound of muscle is also not the same as losing a pound of fat. Losing the muscle slows your metabolism and makes it easier to gain weight, but harder to lose. It also means a larger number of fat cells in your body in proportion to your muscle tissue, leading to an ugly appearance, and even worse, the [dangerous substances](http://www.acs.org/content/acs/en/pressroom/presspacs/2010/acs-presspac-october-13-2010/new-evidence-that-fat-cells-are-not-just-dormant-storage-depots-for-calories.html) that we now know fat cells release into the body.

Fat is associated with heart disease, Type 2 diabetes, and certain cancers. Fat has been found to release a range of hormones and chemicals, some of which have yet to be studied in terms of what they are and what their potential effect could be on your health.

A balanced approach to physical activity is the best way to prevent injury and keep your weight down naturally.

If you have been battering your body with too many high-impact workouts, it's time to take it down a notch or two. If you haven't been working out for a while, it's important to start slowly and sensibly. You can't expect to go from sitting most of your day to doing running marathons.

My wife and I subscribe to a routine of exercising two days and then taking one day off. We just keep cycling through this routine. With both like low-impact activities; she rides a stationary bike while I like an elliptical trainer. We also exercise in our pool by playing a game of water volleyball for 30 minutes during each of the exercise days.

Let's look in the next chapter at the best workouts for those with OA.

Chapter 4 – The Best Workouts For Those With OA

The U.S. Department of Health and Human Services recommends that everyone, including those with arthritis, get 150 minutes of moderate aerobic exercise per week, plus two -30-minute sessions of strength training.

Aerobic exercise

Aerobic exercise raises the heart rate to work the body's most important muscle, the heart. There are many forms of aerobic exercise, but when you have OA, the most important consideration is that it be low impact in order to protect joints.

- Light aerobics
- Aquaerobics
- Walking
- Water walking
- Pilates
- Light calisthenics

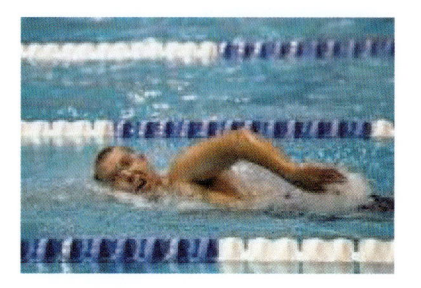

All of these will also improve range of motion, to keep your joints flexible.

A walking program for all

The US Surgeon General has recommended that the easiest way to get your weekly suggested amount of physical activity is to walk 10,000 steps a day, about 3.5 to 5 miles depending on how long your legs and stride are. All you need are some supportive walking shoes and the proper clothing depending on the weather. A pedometer, or a step-counting app for your Smartphone or wearable device like a FitBit can help you keep track of all the steps you do in a day, from your commute to work, to your shopping and housework.

Strength training

Strength training firms muscles, stabilizes joints, and helps prevent injury. Long lean muscle is also more attractive than flab and burns more calories, speeding up your metabolism and making it easier to lose weight.

The weights can be using the machines at the gym, freestanding weights, and/or resistance bands. In terms of OA, the healthiest and safest options are light weights and resistance bands.

Other options for strength training include yoga, tai chi, and functional exercise, that is, focusing on the muscles that you need to perform the most important regular activities in your day, such as carrying your groceries and doing chores around the house.

Yoga and tai chi also improve flexibility and range of motion. In addition, they offer a body, mind and spirit connection through deliberate, meditative movements, not just endless repetitions as you lift weights. Yoga and tai chi also help you become more aware of your body, which can help you avoid injury. In some cases, meditation is even used as a complementary and alternative medicine (CAM) to relieve pain, including the pain of arthritis.

Another way to achieve effective pain relief in relation to OA is to maintain a healthy weight. Let's look at this important topic in the next chapter.

Chapter 5 – Maintaining A Healthy Weight

More than 68% of Americans are now classified as overweight or obese, with the largest percentage now falling into the obese category. This being the case, many people are struggling with OA are probably also struggling with their weight.

Carrying extra weight puts a good deal of additional pressure on joints and the structures that support them, such as tendons and cartilage, causing even more than the usual wear and tear. Studies have shown that for every one pound a person is overweight, they are putting four pounds of additional pressure on their knees when they are walking, and especially when they are going downstairs. So if you are 50 pounds overweight, the extra pressure on your knees is 200 pounds!

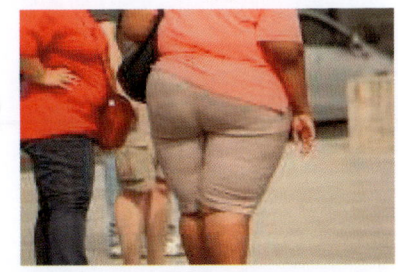

Carrying extra weight affects the entire body all the time. Imagine you are 20 pounds overweight. Now picture yourself carrying four 5-pounds bags of flour with you everywhere as you go through your busy day. Try it as an experiment. You will soon see just how much of a drain it can be on your entire body. When we are standing our entire musculature has to support that weight, including back, hips and knees. If you are sitting, the extra weight will on the back and hip joints.

If we also don't pay attention to our posture, and the way we walk and do other activities, we can cause further damage and uneven wear and tear. For example, women who carry a child or their groceries on one hip rather than in a backpack or a baby carrier at the front are necessarily going to put more weight on one side of the body than the other, leading to uneven wear.

A strong solid set of core muscles will support the back and hips. Good back muscles will prevent lower back pain and injuries such as slipped discs. Good leg muscles will support the knees and hips. Strong leg muscles above and below the knee will support the knees and make them more stable and less prone to injury.

So what is a healthy weight? The Body Mass Index (BMI) (http://www.nhlbi.nih.gov/health/educational/lose_wt/BMI/bmicalc.htm) scale is a useful tool for determining a person's healthy weight based on their height.

It offers a ratio of height to number of pounds and gives a number of different ranges of healthy weight that a person can use as a guideline based on their body type as well.

For example, if we go to a BMI calculator (http://www.nhlbi.nih.gov/health/educational/lose_wt/BMI/bmicalc.htm) and enter the data for a person 5 feet 7 inches tall weighing 180 pounds, the BMI is 28.2. The ranges are:

Underweight = <18.5

Normal weight = 18.5–24.9

Overweight = 25–29.9

Obesity = BMI of 30 or greater

So this person classifies as overweight. If they wanted to get into the normal weight range, they could look at the BMI Tables (http://www.nhlbi.nih.gov/health/educational/lose_wt/BMI/bmi_tbl.htm) to help them determine what a healthy weight would be for their height.

Five feet seven is 67 inches, so a healthy weight according to the table, is between 121 and around 160 pounds.

This gives the person a lot of leeway as to how much weight they would like to lose to get to a healthier weight.

When in doubt, one of the easiest ways to decide how much you should weigh is to look for the middle of the healthy weight range. In this case it would be 140 pounds.

By aiming for the middle range, a person does not have to worry about a few pounds creeping back on and causing them to slip into the overweight category once more. This person would therefore need to set a goal to go down from 180 to 140 pounds through a combination of physical activity and a healthy diet.

It takes 2,000 extra calories consumed to gain a pound, but 3,500 burned to lose one. In round numbers, it is twice as easy to gain weight as to lose it. If you've been struggling with your weight, you're certainly not alone. Fortunately, there are more tools than ever that can help you succeed in losing the weight and keeping it off. We've already discussed the importance of exercise for your OA. Now let's look at a healthy diet in the next chapter.

Chapter 6 – Eating A Healthy, Balanced Diet

You may have heard the old adage "You can't out exercise a bad diet." It is true. Weight loss has to do with 80% diet and 20% exercise. Despite, or perhaps because of, the bountiful food we have in the United States, many Americans struggle with eating a healthy balanced diet. With fast food and convenience foods all around us, it is far too tempting for most people to turn down the food bad for us and opt for smarter food choices.

Most people hear the word diet and think of one lettuce leaf. However, that is not the case. Extreme diets can only lead to more damage to your metabolism and increased weight gain rather than weight loss in the long term.

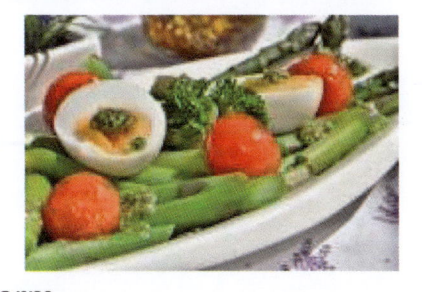

A good diet however, is one rich in natural foods in reasonable portions.

Between calorie control and portion control, and a reasonable amount of exercise each day, most people should be able to lose weight and keep it off no matter what they choose to eat.

One of the most successful diets for both heart health and weight loss is the DASH diet. —DASH stands for Dietary Approaches to Stopping Hypertension, the medical term for high blood pressure. As the name suggests, the theory behind this diet, which was developed by health researchers was to try to lower high blood pressure naturally without resorting to prescription drugs, which usually carry a high risk of unpleasant side effects.

The DASH diet has been clinically proven to not only lower high blood pressure, but also help people lose weight and improve their heart health, and even lower their risk of Type 2 diabetes and certain forms of cancer. Since many people with arthritis also tend to have heart health issues, this might be one of the best places to start if you want to eat a more balanced diet. There is a great deal of free information online to help you get started, with [guidelines](https://www.nhlbi.nih.gov/files/docs/public/heart/dash_brief.pdf) recipes and more to make it as easy as possible for you to lose weight and keep it off.

One of the most popular and heart healthy diet available is the Mediterranean diet. The theory behind this diet is to eat in a similar way to the Italians, Greeks, and other people who lived around the Mediterranean Sea. This diet is rich in plant-based foods such as fresh fruits and vegetables, with small portions of fish and cheese as the protein and very little meat.

Another secret to the Mediterranean eating lifestyle is variety. Studies estimate the Italians eat around 40 to 60 different foods per day.

Many people would agree that Italy has one of the most delicious cuisines in the world. The Italians also have one of the lowest rates of heart disease and obesity. Only 9% of Italians are overweight or obese, compared to 68% of Americans.

Many people worry about their weight for the sake of their appearance. In terms of OA, it is a matter of reducing the wear and tear on your joints and maintaining a heart-healthy lifestyle. Some studies have also suggested that the Mediterranean diet is a good one to follow if you have arthritis due to is anti-inflammatory properties, that is, the ability to reduce irritation in the body. Let's look at following an anti-inflammatory diet in the next chapter.

Chapter 7 – Trying An Anti-Inflammatory Diet

If you've ever suffered from hay fever, you will have a pretty good idea of what inflammation can do to the body, leaving it irritated and uncomfortable or even painful. Some forms of arthritis have an inflammatory component, with red, swollen joints that feel as though they are on fire.

One suggestion for lowering inflammation in the body and improving health is to reduce your stress levels naturally through coping strategies such as meditation and relaxation. Another suggestion is to follow an anti-inflammatory diet.

There are a number of foods suggested can help lower inflammation in the body, and another list of foods to avoid if you wish to lower inflammation.

The exact foods that go into an anti-inflammatory diet have not been established and yet researchers have found that there are foods you can eat that will decrease the inflammation seen in inflammatory arthritis.

Foods found in an anti-inflammatory diet are similar to what is seen in the Mediterranean diet, which has a large amount of vegetables, fish, and olive oil in the diet. The Zone diet is also an example of an anti-inflammation diet.

The actual foods in an anti-inflammatory diet differ depending on whom you ask but in general, the recommendations are these:

- Eat low amounts of trans fats and saturated fats.

- Eat a lot of fruits and vegetables.

- Eat plenty of foods that are high in omega 3 fatty acids, such as fish and walnuts.

- Decrease the intake of white rice and pasta, which are high in refined carbohydrates.

- Choose whole grains, such as wheat bread and brown rice.

- Choose spices that have anti-inflammatory properties, such as curry and ginger.

- Avoid highly processed or refined foods and instead make food from scratch.

- Select lean meat sources, such as poultry, avoiding red meat and dairy products that are high in fat.

Eating an anti-inflammatory diet doesn't necessarily mean you'll lose weight but most people do lose some weight on this type of diet. This takes the pressure off the joints and reduces the pain and inflammation of arthritis.

Best Foods to Eat

While there isn't any dietary cure for arthritis, there are some foods that have been found to be beneficial against inflammation, increase the effectiveness of the immune system, and make bones stronger. The following foods are considered good to take in if you have arthritis:

- **Fish.** Fish are high in omega 3 fatty acids, which are anti-inflammatory. You should eat at least two servings of fish per week, such as herring, mackerel, tuna, and salmon. Fish is especially good for rheumatoid arthritis.

- **Oils.** Certain oils, such as extra virgin olive oil are beneficial because they contain healthy fats and nutrients such as oleocanthal. Oleocanthal provides for decreases in inflammation, similar to that found in non-steroidal anti-inflammatory medications. You can also choose avocado oil or safflower oil that lower cholesterol. Oils are good for osteoarthritis and rheumatoid arthritis.

- **Soy products.** Soy products such as edamame and tofu are high in omega 3 fatty acids, fiber, and protein. Soy products are excellent food to eat if you have rheumatoid arthritis.

- **Cherries.** Cherries are especially good for gouty arthritis. They are high in anthocyanins, which are anti-inflammatory by nature. You can find anthocyanins in raspberries, strawberries, blackberries, and blueberries.

- **Broccoli.** Broccoli is good for osteoarthritis because it is high in vitamin C, vitamin K, and sulforaphane, which has found to be a good choice in the prevention and progression of osteoarthritis. Broccoli is high in calcium, which fights osteoporosis.

- **Dairy products.** Dairy products that are low in fat can help fight osteoarthritis and osteoporosis. They are high in vitamin D and calcium, which increase the strength of the bones. Dairy products enhance the immune system. If you don't like dairy, you can get your calcium and vitamin D by eating leafy green vegetables.

- **Green tea.** Green tea is high in polyphenols, which are antioxidants that have been shown to decrease inflammation and to slow the progression of cartilage breakdown.

Green tea is also high in EGCG (epigallocatechin-3-gallate), which is effective against those substances that damage the joints in rheumatoid arthritis.

- **Citrus fruits.** These are good for arthritis because they are high in vitamin C, which prevents inflammation in patients with osteoarthritis and rheumatoid arthritis. Good citrus fruits include lemons, oranges, limes, and grapefruits.

- **Beans.** Beans are high in fiber, which naturally decreases the level of C-reactive protein—a protein that results in inflammation. Beans are also high in minerals and folic acid, which help stimulate the immune system and fight rheumatoid arthritis. Red beans, such as pinto beans and kidney beans, are the best choices for arthritis.

- **Whole grains.** Whole grains also decrease the levels of C-reactive protein in the bloodstream. C-reactive protein helps reduce the amount of inflammation found in conditions like diabetes, heart disease, and rheumatoid arthritis. Try getting whole grains by eating whole grain cereal, brown rice, and oatmeal, which are high in rheumatoid arthritis.

- **Garlic.** Garlic, leaks, and onions are part of the allium family, which decreases symptoms in osteoarthritis.

Scientists believe that diallyl disulphine in garlic will decrease the amount of enzymes in the joint that damage cartilage. Garlic is especially good for osteoarthritis.

- **Nuts.** Nuts have high levels of alpha linolenic acid (ALA), minerals, vitamin E, fiber, and protein. The best nuts to choose are pistachios, almonds, pine nuts, and almonds. Nuts help you lose weight, which benefits the joints in all types of arthritis.

Other foods to try include:

- Salmon and Other Fatty Fish with Omega-3s
- Probiotics, that is, yogurt with live cultured, or pickled foods such as pickled vegetables
- Olive Oil
- Cherries
- Peppers, such as red, green and yellow ones
- Ginger
- Turmeric
- Green leafy vegetables and cruciferous vegetables
- Berries such as blueberries

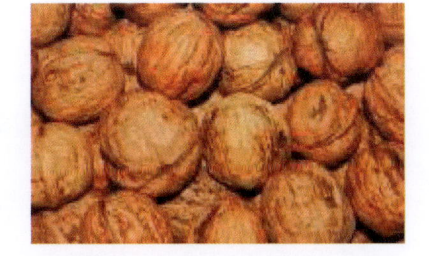

As we can see from the list of anti-inflammatory foods, many of them are part of a Mediterranean diet, with the exception of ginger and turmeric, which are popular Indian spices.

Foods To Avoid

There are some foods that actually increase inflammation. Foods you need to avoid if you have arthritis include the following:

- **Trans fats.** Trans fats damage the lining of the blood vessels, inducing inflammation. Because trans fats are mainly manmade, we don't break them down very easily so the end result is inflammation of the joints.

- **White bread and pasta.** These break down into simple sugars that lead to inflammation. Inflammatory markers are higher in those people who eat processed wheat foods, so there is more joint pain and inflammation in arthritic patients.

- **Saturated fats.** Saturated fats are high in arachidonic acid that causes inflammation. Instead of saturated fats, you need to eat more unsaturated fats, which don't lead to inflammation. Saturated fats are found in red meats as well as in high-fat dairy products.

- **Omega 6 fatty acids.** These can be found in some types of seeds. If you are going to eat fatty foods, make sure that the balance is toward omega 3 fatty acids and lower in omega 6 fatty acids.

- **MSG.** Foods that are preserved in monosodium glutamate (MSG) can increase the level of inflammation in the body. This is why it is better to make your own food from scratch so you can avoid foods that might be preserved with MSG.

- **Gluten.** Even if you don't have celiac disease, you should decrease the amount of gluten in your diet. Gluten isn't inflammatory in everyone but may be the cause of some of the inflammation you are experiencing.

Other foods to avoid include:

- Sugar
- Salt
- Standard Cooking Oils
- Red Meat
- Processed Meats/Cold Cuts
- Artificial Sweeteners and Flavorings
- Alcohol

- Full-fat Dairy Products

In terms of the inflammatory foods, many of them are part of an unhealthy Western diet, particularly the trans fats in fast foods and cakes, cookies and other snacks that are found on supermarket shelves. While we should try to lower our intake of saturated fat and increase the unsaturated type, we MUST avoid trans fat altogether. In most cases it is a manufactured fat and the body doesn't know how to get rid of it as it does with "natural" fats, so it stores it as fat.

Refined carbohydrates and other foods with glutens in them irritates peoples' system with celiac disease, a severe gastrointestinal disorder. Many people going gluten-free report feeling much better overall in only a few short days.

If you are feeling run down, achy, or stiff, try cutting back on the inflammatory foods and adding some of the delicious anti-inflammatory foods to your diet, and see what a difference it can make to your health.

Chapter 8 – Improving Joint Mobility And Stability

We have already discussed the importance of exercise for your OA, but working out should not be your only focus. There are a number of ways to improve joint mobility, flexibility and stability.

Stretching

Slow, gentle stretching of joints may improve flexibility, lessen stiffness and reduce pain. Exercises such as yoga and tai chi are great ways to manage stiffness. Warming up and cooling down before any workout can also help, and in addition, protects from injury.

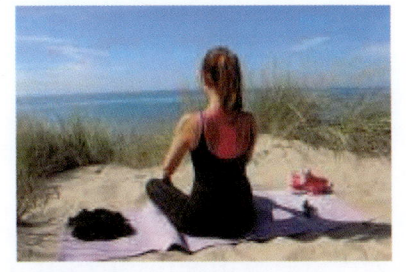

Keeping your muscles warm

Cold muscles tend to be tense and tight, leaving them prone to injury (and pain – cold damp environments increases my joint pain substantially). The joints will also stiffen, therefore losing range of motion and flexibility. Avoid working out in a cold room and cover yourself after you work out.

For example, you can put on a hoodie and sweat pants over your workout clothes when you are done. When it is time to do deep meditation in yoga, many people find a blanket to be very helpful.

In relation to yoga, there are a number of props that can improve your practice. These include cushions to sit on or to support different poses, plus blocks and straps. Each are intended to avoid injury and make it easier to get into the poses and maintain them. A [strap](http://amzn.to/1sflmfn) (http://amzn.to/1sflmfn) can increase flexibility as it allows you to deepen the pose little by little and gradually stretch more.

Water workouts

Workouts in a pool with reasonably warm (not cold) water can do wonders for your mobility. It is low impact but high resistance, since your muscles need to do their work against the pressure of the water. Water walking, weight lifting and water aerobics and calisthenics will all give you a good workout and make a nice change from your usual routine. After water volleyball, we usually do either an upper body workout using [aqua barbells](http://amzn.to/1P3I8Rj) (http://amzn.to/1P3I8Rj) or a lower body workout.

Warm showers and baths

If you don't have a pool near you, not to worry. A warm shower or bath can ease tight muscles and allow for deeper stretches. If you are working out at home, start with a shower and finish your session with a shower or bath and see what a difference it can make to your joint pain from OA. A 20-minute soak in a hot tub with 102 degree Fahrenheit water or spa works wonders for my OA joint pain.

All of your efforts still might not be enough to keep your joints flexible and stable. In this case, assistive devices might be called for. Let's look at this topic in the next chapter.

Chapter 9 – Using Assistive Devices

If you are really struggling with arthritis pain, discuss assistive device options with your doctor. They will then give you a referral to a physical or occupational therapist. They understand body dynamics and pain relief, and can provide a range of treatment options for pain management including:

- Ways to properly use joints
- Assistive devices
- Heat and cold therapies
- Range of motion and flexibility exercises

We will discuss the latter 2 options in a moment. Let's focus for the moment on assistive devices.

There are a number of assistive devices that can offer support to joints affected by OA and prevent further wear and tear, or injury to the joint.

Assistive devices can help with function and mobility. They range from simple tools to make life easier, to items that can maintain mobility even in the face of severe disability.

Handy tools include:

- Arthritis gloves
- Jar openers
- Long-handled grippers for reaching up high to grasp items such as cereal boxes
- Easy-grip scissors
- Easy grip cutlery
- Long-handled shoe horns
- Steering wheel grips
- Velcro-fastened clothing and shoes
- Hand rails for homes
- Stair lifts for multiple-storied houses
- Raised toilet seats with handles to make it easier to get up and down

Mobility devices include:

- Braces
- Splits
- Shoe orthotics
- Canes

- Walkers

- Scooters

- Wheelchairs

- Motorized wheelchairs

Many of these items can be found at pharmacies and medical supply stores and are often covered by insurance. Certain items, such as custom knee braces or orthotics, will usually have to be prescribed by a doctor and are fitted by a physical or occupational therapist. They can be very expensive and not always covered by insurance, so be sure to discuss all of your options with your doctor if your budget is tight.

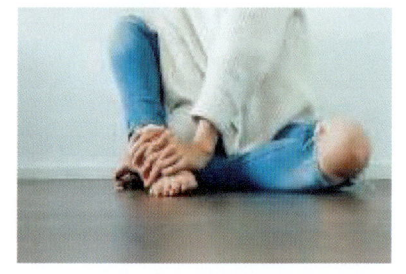

Assistive devices can provide pain relief because you are straining less. Best of all, they are pill-free ways to help your OA pain. There are many other ways to get OA pain relief without popping pills. Let's look at complementary and alternative therapies in the next chapter.

Chapter 10 – Using Complementary And Alternative Therapies

When you are in the throes of pain, all you want is relief. For most, this means reaching for an over-the-counter painkiller. Others prefer to find pill-free pain relief but aren't sure where to find it. There are a number of complementary and alternative therapies (CAM), some of them thousands of years old, and covered by most insurance companies. Below are some options you may want to consider the next time you're in pain.

Acupuncture is a form of therapy used in traditional Chinese medicine, which is centuries old. Very thin, sterile needles are placed just under the skin on specific points of the body. Studies show that acupuncture is effective in treating up to 100 conditions including chronic pain. While acupuncture hasn't always been accepted in Western medicine, more doctors have referred patients to acupuncturists than any other "alternative" medicine available today.

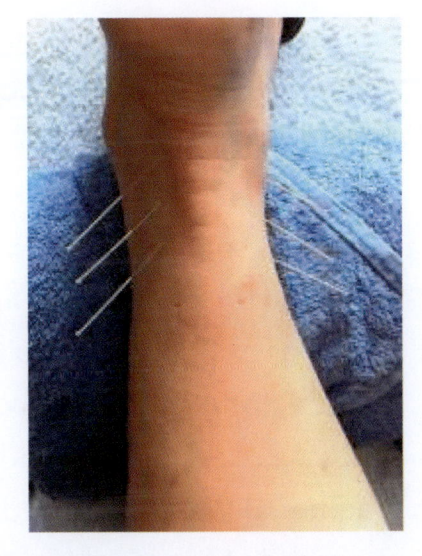

Acupressure works in a similar way, but without the needles. The energy centers that the acupuncturists would normally place needles on are instead pressed.

Massage therapy is another natural form of pain relief for every part of the body, from head to toe. Just think about it - when you have a headache, you often rub the aching area, such as the temples, bridge of the nose between the sinuses, and/or the back of the neck. In the same way, licensed massage therapists can relieve aches and pains through the skill in their hand and their knowledge of human physiology.

Acupressure and massage therapy can be used in conjunction with aromatherapy. [Aromatherapy (https://www.amazon.com/Aromatherapy-Science-Relaxation-Essential-Response-ebook/dp/B0108T4DTQ)](https://www.amazon.com/Aromatherapy-Science-Relaxation-Essential-Response-ebook/dp/B0108T4DTQ) as the name suggests, helps heal through the aroma of plant extracts, which are known as essential oils. They don't just smell great, however. Essential oils have powerful therapeutic qualities as well, to help relieve pain. For example, birch oil is the source of aspirin, so if you are not allergic to it, you can use it as part of a pain-relieving massage. Aromatherapy is an essential part of traditional Indian (Ayurvedic) medicine, which is thousands of years old.

Both traditional Chinese medicine and Ayurvedic medicine also use herbs and supplements to relieve arthritis pain. Let's look at a few of your options in the next chapter.

Chapter 11 - Herbs and Supplements

Traditional medical texts from Ayurvedic and traditional Chinese medicine show that people have used herbs to treat pain for thousands of years. For those concerned about the side effects of over the counter and prescription medications, certain herbs and supplements might provide relief from your OA pain. They can be consumed on their own, added to food in some cases, or applied to the skin in various ways.

Herbs

Herbs known to offer relief from arthritis pain include:
- Ginger
- Turmeric
- Chili powder
- Rosemary

Ginger can be drunk as a tasty tea or added to a stir fry. The first three seasonings are delicious in Indian dishes. Rosemary is a good seasoning for chicken or roasted vegetables.

Supplements

Supplements used in capsule form to relieve OA pain include:
- arnica

- black cohosh
- dandelion
- devil's claw
- feverfew
- juniper
- meadowsweet
- white willow

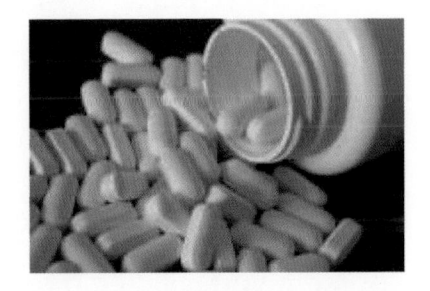

Remember, just because these items are natural does not mean they are completely without side effects, so be sure to read details about each one carefully before you start to take it.

Topical uses

Some of these herbs are used as salves, poultices, or additives to a warm tub of water. Japanese volcanic bath salts also work well. Add to a tub of hot water and allow to dissolve. Get into the water when you can tolerate it, and soak for at least 10 minutes or until the water starts to cool.

There are several other natural ways to manage your OA symptoms. Let's look at a few of these in the next chapter.

Chapter 12 – Managing Symptoms, Such As Pain, Stiffness and Swelling

Sometimes, no matter how well you take care of yourself, you will begin to feel aches and pains from your OA. However, your lifestyle can greatly influence the symptoms you feel, and the severity of the pain. There are several lifestyle measures that can help you manage the pain, stiffness and swelling of OA.

Be aware of your posture as you sit, stand and walk. Proper posture can make a huge difference in preventing unneeded stress on your spine and lower back. It also reduces neck strain and pain in your hips and knees.

If you spend much time on the computer, in addition to being aware of your posture, consider the placement of your keyboard. Move it forward, closer to your body, to reduce strain on your shoulders, arms and neck. Using a keyboard rest, orthopedic chair that offers good support, a foot wedge, and other supportive devices might also make your time in front of the computer less damaging to your joints. A lifetime of wear and tear can all start to add up if we are not careful.

Don't spend too much time sitting. If you work at a sedentary job, get up from your desk at least every three hours – sooner if possible. Even if you can't go for a little walk, stand up to stretch or bend over to touch your toes. Ease yourself into whatever movement you chose, and don't bounce. Doing some type of stretching throughout the day will keep you less stiff and more supple.

As we have mentioned, carrying extra weight can cause joint pain, or aggravate it.

Exercises such as walking, swimming or water aerobics, yoga and cycling exercises don't put undue stress on your joints and also release endorphins that ease pain as well as improve your mood. There's no need to spend hours working out in the gym. Research has shown that only 30 minutes of exercise each day can ease the pain of arthritis, and even those 30 minutes can be broken up into 10 minute sessions and be just as effective as working out in one large chunk of time.

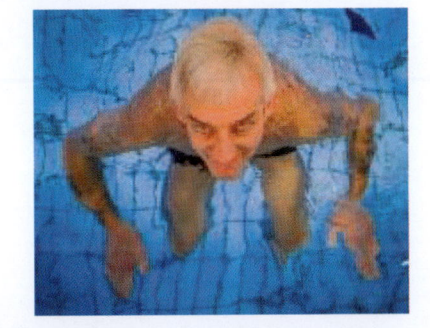

Hot or cold therapy can be used to treat arthritis pain. Normally either an ice pack or a bag of frozen vegetables wrapped in a towel, or a heating pad, is placed on the painful area. It is important to remove the treatment after 20 minutes, but it can be repeated two to three times daily.

Some people use Icy Hot and similar patches, but they can cause skin irritation and are expensive. And like many over the counter remedies, they can have side effects. Let's look at over the counter medications used to treat OA in the next chapter.

Chapter 13 – Over The Counter Medications

There are a number of standard over the counter medications that offer pain relief for those with OA. They include:

Nonsteroidal anti-inflammatory drugs (NSAIDs)

These are the most commonly used drugs to ease inflammation and related pain. NSAIDs include aspirin and ibuprofen. They are generally considered safe unless you have an allergy, but can cause gastrointestinal bleeding over time. That was the issue I had with them and had to give them up.

Analgesics

These pain relievers include acetaminophen, the brand name of which is Tylenol. Tylenol is used in more than 140 different over the counter and prescription medicines, ranging from pain reliever to cold medicines and more. It is important to read all labels and follow dosing instructions to the letter to avoid accidental overdose and damage to the liver.

Topical pain relievers

These can include creams, gels, lotions and patches designed to relieve pain. Popular choices include Aspercreme, with aspirin in it (so avoid if allergic) and Capzasin cream and patches, which use the essence of red chili peppers to provide pain relief.

Chapter 14 – Prescription Medications

There are a number of prescription medications used to treat OA pain. Two of the most common are:

- Naproxen
- Celecoxib

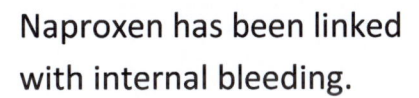

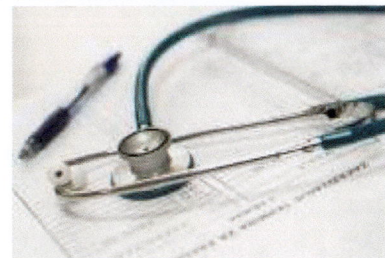

Naproxen has been linked with internal bleeding. Celecoxib is safe and effective, however, it is not as widely prescribed as perhaps it ought to be because several other drugs in the same class (COX-2 inhibitors) were taking off the market several years ago because of concerns over how they affected the heart.

For heavy duty-pain relief, there are

- Opioids (narcotics)
- Tramadol (Ultram) (an atypical opioid)

However, there are increasing concerns about them being addictive.

Patches

Fentanyl patches can offer powerful pain relief right at the site of the pain. They do pose a risk of side effects, however, so should be used exactly as directed.

Corticosteroids

Corticosteroids are powerful anti-inflammatory medicines taken by mouth or injected directly into a joint at a doctor's office. They are effective, but carry a range of serious side effects. Steroid injections provide OA relief, but there is a limit to how often you can have them.

Hyaluronic acid

Hyaluronic acid occurs naturally in joint fluid, acting as a shock absorber and lubricant for your joints. However, the acid appears to break down in people with osteoarthritis. The injections are done in a doctor's office and should last several months, to protect the joint and ease pain. These provide relief, but can't be used too often.

As you have seen, there are many different strategies for getting OA pain relief, but one of the best ways to deal with it can be to maintain a healthy mindset. Let's look at this topic in the next chapter.

Chapter 15 – Maintaining A Positive And Healthy Mindset

Whenever a person has a chronic illness such as OA, it is important for them to have a positive outlook. Those that do remain positive tend to take better care of themselves. Those who suffer from depression and anxiety do not look after themselves as well, so tend to have poorer outcomes.

Up to 50% of seniors can experience depression at some stage, and up to 75% of people who have heart disease. If you have both arthritis and heart disease, you should pay particular attention to your mental health and well-being.

Stress relief techniques are important for everyone, but those with stiff joints could do without the tensing of the muscles triggered by stressful situations. Making time for yourself to do something you enjoy, such as take a long soak in a warm tub, can refresh body and mind.

There are other-mind and body techniques that can be used specifically to treat pain without resorting to pills. These include:

- Relaxation

- Biofeedback

- Guided imagery

- Journaling, especially keeping a pain journal in relation to your OA

- Meditation

- Yoga with meditation

- Tai chi-deep breathing and meditative movement

- Praying, engaging in religious study

- Joining a support group, online or in person

... and more.

If you stop taking an interest in your usual activities, or in trying to live as normal a life as possible despite your OA, it could be a sign of depression. Body, mind and spirit are all connected, so do not underestimate the effect of OA on your mood and try to remain positive.

If you still struggle, consider finding a therapist or joining a support group. Don't underestimate the value of learning more about your condition as well. New research is coming out all the time on OA, which could mean even more new options for your OA pain relief.

However, if all of the above-mentioned techniques still do not give you sufficient pain relief, or there is just too much damage to an essential joint like a knee or hip, it may be time to consider surgery.

Chapter 16 – Considering Surgical Options

Every form of surgery carries with it some degree of risk, but in the case of OA, there are quite a few pros and cons and it is important to note that the new artificial joint will most definitely not be the same as your natural one.

Having said that, if your mobility and quality of life are seriously impaired by your OA in the knee or hip, it may be time to consider replacement surgery. This is a huge decision, and one you need to research carefully in order to be as informed as possible about what to expect. In particular, getting ready before the surgery, and understanding everything that will be involved in the recovery time is essential to try to get the best results.

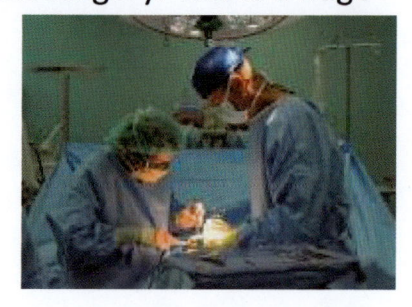

For example, everyone will need physical therapy and rehabilitation after joint replacement surgery. But some studies have shown that those who do 'pre-habilitation', that is, structured exercises prior to the surgery, tend to have a better outcome.

Getting ready with the practical aspects of being laid up for weeks is also important, especially if you live alone. Packing the freezer with healthy, low calorie meals you have made yourself and can just heat and eat will help maintain a high level of nutrition without too many calories being consumed, in order to prevent weight gain while you are recuperating.

No one likes to think about having surgery, but if your doctor suggests it, and you have exhausted all other forms of treatment, be sure to learn all you can about joint replacement surgery. Also consider your overall health and any other existing medical conditions, and then make an informed decision.

Conclusion

In this guide, you have discovered a range of ways to take control of your OA to relieve pain and inflammation and limit the impact on your quality of life. You have learned about preventing arthritis and managing OA through a number of effective measures, including:

- getting enough exercise/physical activity
- using common sense in relation to working out to prevent or manage your OA
- the best workouts for OA
- maintaining a healthy weight
- eating a healthy diet
- trying an anti-inflammatory diet
- improving joint mobility, flexibility and stability
- using assistive devices
- using complementary and alternative therapies
- herbs and supplements
- managing symptoms, such as pain, stiffness and swelling

- over the counter medications
- prescription medications
- maintaining a positive and healthy mindset
- considering surgical options

Trying one or more of these can not only help with your OA, they should also be able to add to your overall well-being, especially exercising, watching your weight, and eating a healthy diet.

One thing is for sure-doing nothing about your OA is not an option, because it will only get worse if you don't take sensible steps for self-care. Here's to your best self even with OA, independent and mobile!

Resources

What is Osteoarthritis?

http://www.arthritis.org/about-arthritis/types/osteoarthritis/

WebMD OA Health Center

http://www.webmd.com/osteoarthritis/guide/osteoarthritis-treatment-care

Mayo Clinic

http://www.mayoclinic.org/diseases-conditions/osteoarthritis/basics/treatment/con-20014749

Best Foods for Arthritis

http://www.arthritis.org/living-with-arthritis/arthritis-diet/best-foods-for-arthritis/best-foods-for-arthritis.php

The Mediterranean Diet

http://www.mayoclinic.org/healthy-lifestyle/nutrition-and-healthy-eating/in-depth/mediterranean-diet/art-20047801

Other Senior Health and Fitness Books by This Author

If you would like to read more about Senior Health and Fitness, here is a list of the titles, CreateSpace links and descriptions:

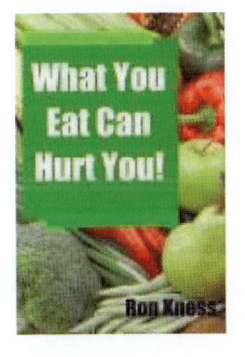

What You Eat Can Hurt You

https://www.createspace.com/4963196

Do you know that certain foods increase your risk for inflammation, disease and illness? It's true! And certain foods can help cure and heal you if you do get sick. Knowing which foods to eat and which ones to avoid empowers you to manage your own health.

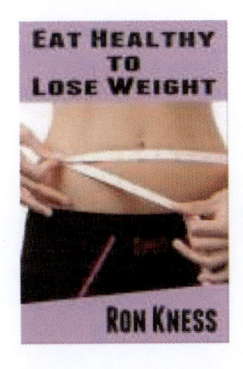

Eat Healthy to Lose Weight

https://www.createspace.com/4962939

As you read through our book, we show you which foods you should and should not be eating to reach your weight loss goal, along with discussing how to maintain your weight loss and stay within a few pounds of your goal weight. Banish the weight you keep gaining back each time by learning how to live a healthy lifestyle.

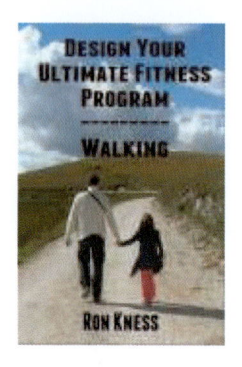

Design Your Ultimate Fitness Program - Walking

https://www.createspace.com/5252272

In my book Design Your Ultimate Fitness Program – Walking, we discuss the considerations that need to be made when designing a custom walking program, along with:
• Equipment needed
• Wearable technology you can use to track your walking
• And how to make walking more challenging

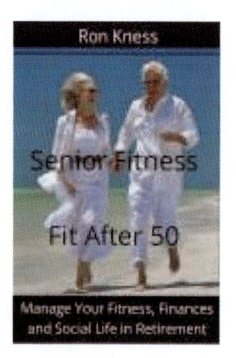

Senior Fitness – Fit After 50: Learn How to Manage Your Fitness, Finances and Social Life in Retirement

https://www.createspace.com/5474751

Inside you will discover answers to your most pressing questions:
• What do I need to know about downsizing my home?
• What are the best tips for staying healthy as you approach your 50's?
• When should I start planning for retirement?
• I am worried about being lonely once I retire, do others feel the same?
• Is it worthwhile to carry two homes during retirement?
And more…

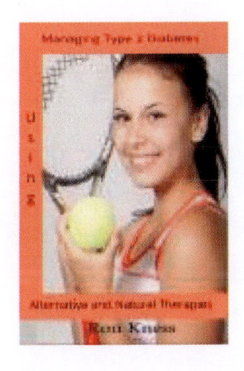

Managing Type 2 Diabetes Using Alternative And Natural Therapies

https://www.createspace.com/5401244

While Type 2 diabetes can be managed medically, there are many alternative natural and holistic methods of therapy and treatment that can further enhance quality of life and minimize the effects of this disease. In this book, I discuss 12 different types, including yoga, reflexology and acupuncture to name just three.

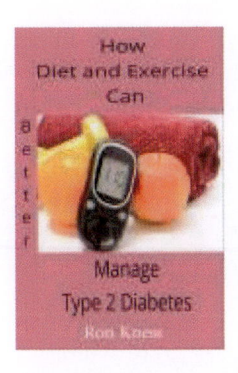

How Diet and Exercise Can Better Manage Type 2 Diabetes

https://www.createspace.com/5404845

Of the different types of diabetes, only Type 2 can be reversed. In my book How Diet and Exercise Can Better Manage Type 2 Diabetes, we reveal the three things you can do to best manage your disease, including:
• Diet
• Exercise
• Weight management

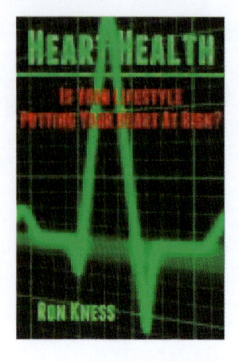

Heart Health: Is Your Lifestyle Putting Your Heart at Risk?

https://www.createspace.com/5464020

In my ebook Is Your Lifestyle Putting Your Heart At Risk? we discuss the six greatest risks to your heart and the lifestyle changes you can make to mitigate them.

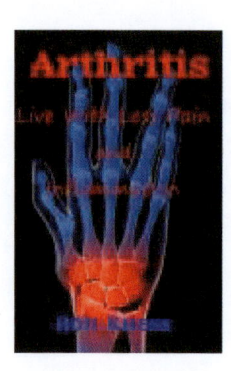

Arthritis – Live Wth Less Pain and Inflammation: Tips and Techniques You Can Use to Lessen the Pain and Inflammation

https://www.createspace.com/5457441

Discover Simple Tips & Information That Will Help Reduce The Painful Symptoms Of Arthritis!

You learn things like:
• Simple and effective information that will help you manage the pain and inflammation that comes along with arthritis, so that you can live an active, full life without debilitating pain.
• The different types of arthritis, their symptoms and how to alleviate their painful side effects.
• The pros and cons of over-the-counter arthritis medications, plus simple tips that will help you know how to choose the right supplements.
• Free, yet effective ways to get relief from arthritis pain and inflammation, so you don't have to suffer anymore.

the effects arthritis can have significant impact on your physical and mental well-being, but this books shows you how to overcome its painful symptoms and live life relatively pain free.

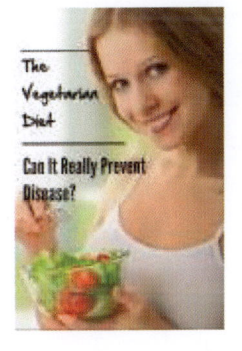

The Vegetarian Diet – Can It Really Prevent Disease?

https://www.createspace.com/5519874

Is a vegetarian diet right for you? Multiple studies have shown over and over that a vegetarian diet goes along way in preventing certain chronic diseases, such as:

- Heart Disease
- Cancer
- Diverticulitis
- Type 2 Diabetes
- Hypertension
- Obesity
- Kidney Failure

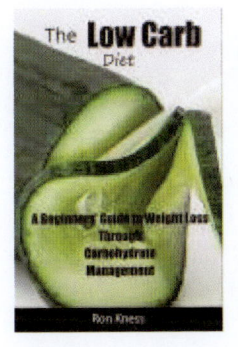

The Low Carb Diet: A Beginner's Guide to Weight Loss Through Carbohydrate Management

https://www.createspace.com/5416348

In my book "The Low-Carb Diet – A Beginners' Guide to Weight Loss Through Carbohydrate Management", I reveal a successful method of losing weight based in part on the amount and type of carbohydrates you consume.

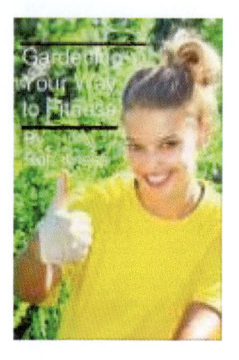

[Gardening Your Way to Fitness: The Fun Way to Get Fit and Provide Beauty and Healthful Bounty for Your Family](https://www.createspace.com/5459564)

https://www.createspace.com/5459564

The gym is a great place to stay fit during the colder seasons, but once the temperature turns warmer you want to spend more time outside. Plus, you'll have the benefit of fresh wholesome produce to enjoy by growing vegetables in your backyard garden.

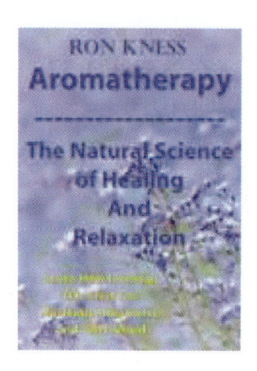

[Aromatherapy - The Science of Healing and Relaxation: Learn How Essential Oils Elicit The Relaxation Response And Alter Mood](https://www.createspace.com/5714434)

https://www.createspace.com/5714434

In my book Aromatherapy – The Science of Healing and Relaxation, we reveal the natural holistics methods you can use to heal the body from certain medical issues and to relive stress through relaxation. In particular we talk about:
• Aromatherapy - what it is and how it works
• Essential Oils – how the effects of certain aromas differs from others
• Recipes – how to make your own essential oil combinations

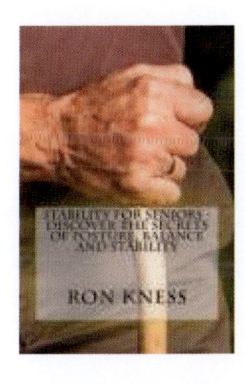

[Stability for Seniors](): [Discover the Secrets of Posture, Balance and Stability]()

https://www.createspace.com/6096479

Many people sacrifice their health in pursuit of their career. They are so busy making a living that they neglect to make a life. The excuse that they do not have time to exercise is tossed about so frequently that they end up letting their health and fitness slide.

If you are not regularly active, you will have muscular atrophy over time. Your flexibility will decrease. Your core strength will diminish. As time progresses, you will be less limber and more rigid.

This is exactly how people age poorly. It's a process that has snowballed over time.

Only with regular exercise and a healthy diet can you have a body that is fit and has the ability to almost reverse aging.

If you have neglected your health for years and life seems to be a chore now because you can't get around without assistance, do not feel dejected.

You can remedy the situation. You can restore the strength, balance and stamina that you have lost. It is never too late to become what you might have been.

This guide will show you exactly what you need to do to restore your balance, strengthen your core and give you the ability to live life to its fullest. Read how …

About The Author

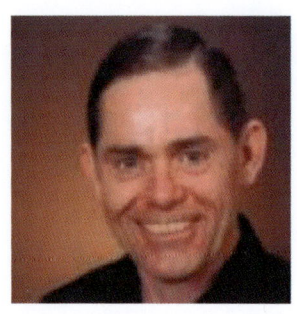

Besides my own writing, I also ghostwrite ebooks, reports, articles, blogs and do Kindle conversions for my clients on a variety of topics.

Today my wife and I live in Gold Canyon, AZ, where you'll find me happily sitting in my office typing away on my laptop as I work on my next book or ghostwriting project . . . that is if we are not traveling on a cruise ship - our new-found mode of travel.

If you like my book, please leave a review of it.

Printed in Great Britain
by Amazon